When the Scheresky family learned that Ted, in the prime of his life, was the victim of a rapidly spreading cancer, their happy family life turned into a nightmare of disbelief and despair. Displaying unrelenting courage and uplifting faith through the last tender, painful days of Ted's life, the family trusted God's promise that He would work out His very best in His plans for their lives. We all can identify with the human struggle to accept terminal illness, the death of a loved one and the practical problems one faces when the head of the family dies. Let Jeanne Scheresky show you how the Christian love that surrounded her family and their own deeply rooted faith strengthened them and helped them to pass through the valley of their despair and emerge victorious.

Diagnosis: CANCER

where do we go from here?

Jeanne Scheresky

New Life Ventures

MARSHALL, MORGAN & SCOTT

LONDON

NEW LIFE VENTURES
Marshall, Morgan & Scott
a member of the Pentos Group
1 Bath Street, London EC1V 9LB

First Published in the United States of America
by Fleming H. Revell Company 1977
First published in Great Britain by
Marshall, Morgan & Scott 1978

ISBN 0 551 05578 2

Printed in Great Britain by Cox & Wyman Ltd,
London, Reading and Fakenham

8720 R01

TO Mama and Papa—Ted's parents

It was their love, influence, and example that helped create the very special man with whom I shared twenty-two years of my life . . . for which I will always be grateful.

Contents

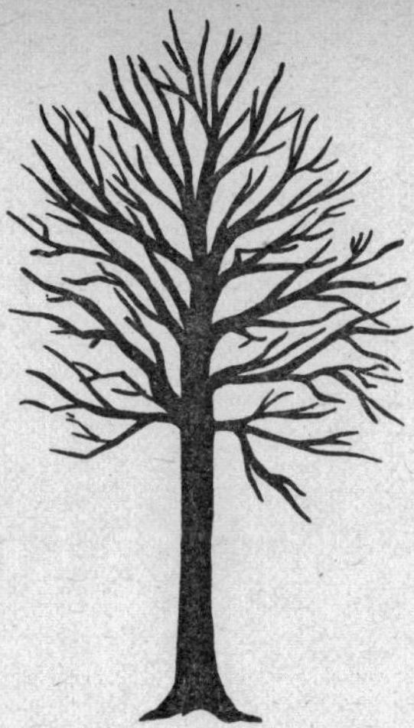

This bare oak tree is a symbol of a life that is left alone, stripped of all that is good and worthwhile and dear—lonely, empty, and dead.

I want it to remind me, not of the pain and anguish that we shared on the path God led us along, but of the comfort of His loving arms around us . . . . Not to hug my grief to my heart in self-pity, but to remind me of God's sufficiency in the face of desolation.

As the oak tree blooms anew each spring, so I have faith that God will someday bring springtime to my heart and life again. But I never want to be so happy that I forget these long, dark, painful days, when I proved God's promises are true.

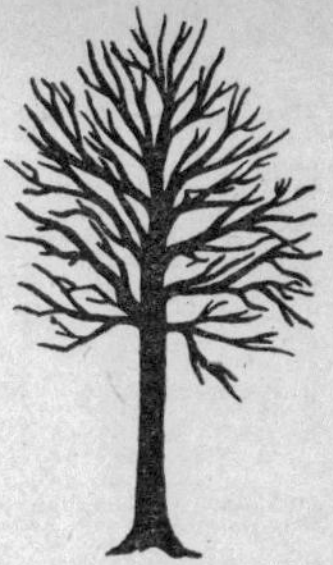

1

Turbulence and Tears

What are *feelings?* Sensations? Hot and cold? Emotions? Joy, sadness, elation, despair?

Fear? *Fear,* resulting in a pounding heart that slides up into your throat and threatens to choke off your breathing. Sweat trickling down your back between your shoulder blades. Legs made of poor-quality rubber. Knees of melted Jell-O. Numb lips, which you find difficult to use to form words. Words that stumble over themselves, not really communicating the idea that is crashing confusingly through your weary mind. Thoughts racing, leaping across the miles, whirling like a child's toy top until the pictures of Mickey Mouse become a blur of yellow, red, and blue as it goes faster and faster.

My mind leaped across the 1300 miles of frozen mountains and prairie to North Dakota and my darling Ted, the children, our home, our happy life together. It jerked back to where I stood in a little town in Oregon, beside a hospital bed that held my dear, terribly ill mother.

Feelings? Disbelief, unreality—this must be some horrible joke, a bad dream. But in the fraction of a minute that it took to feel all of this, my mind was also accepting the fact that Dr. Larson *was* on the phone. He was an excellent doctor. A trusted friend for over twenty years, he wouldn't call me clear from North Dakota without a very good reason.

When the phone rang that bright, sunny, spring morning, I got it on the first ring, as it was on a low table at the foot of the hospital bed in my mother's living room. She was not sleeping, as I had just bathed her and gotten her ready for the day, but she was very sick, and I knew that the shrillness of the phone was grating to her. In my wildest imaginings I could not have dreamed how my life would be changed by picking up that ordinary black telephone! The voice came quickly to the point. "Jean, this is Dr. Larson. Ted just left my office. I want you to sit down. I have bad news for you."

I pulled a chair over with my foot and perched on the edge. I can remember the physical feeling of my face smiling as my mind raced ahead to the possibilities. It wouldn't be Lorie, our nineteen-year-old son. He was in Lincoln, Nebraska, in college. But it flitted across my consciousness: "Oh, if he broke his leg again, I'll have five months of bathing a six-foot-two boy who is sitting on the edge of the tub with one leg in a long, dirty, smelly cast, the other in the tub. There'll be moanings and complaints of 'You have too much soap on the rag. Look out, you are getting water on the cast!' "

I doubted it would be Jody. It was the wrong time of the year for falling out of hay mows. It was too cold for falling off a horse. It couldn't be her!

My mind raced on to Ted. It *couldn't* be him; he had a complete physical the week before I left. He had never been sick in his life, before the previous August. He developed a terrible pain in his back one day when he and his brother Jim were on their way into Minot. As it was harvest time, Jim merely dropped Ted off at the hospital and went on with his errands, planning to pick up Ted on the way back.

Ted found Dr. Larson, who popped him in bed and diagnosed the pain as a kidney-stone attack, accompanied by excruciating pain—unrelenting, unbelievable, searing, red-hot pain. With three attacks in two days, plus X-rays and tests, once the pain stopped, Ted was anxious to get on with the harvest. Dr. Larson concluded that his original diagnosis was correct and let Ted go home.

By November, Ted was feeling terribly tired all of the time, but decided that it was just old age creeping up on him. He was working three jobs a day. He was up at 5:00 A.M. to feed cattle, driving the school bus for a neighbor who had lost his leg in a hay baler during the summer, and wiring a house for some friends. Then it was back to run the bus, home for chores in the dark, and often supper was not till 8:00 or 8:30 at night.

He was forty-five—he deserved to be tired! In all of our twenty-two years of marriage, he hadn't been sick; he had stomachaches in the spring and fall from the tensions of waltzing with the weather, trying to get the crops seeded and harvested. What could it be, that would cause Dr. Larson to call me clear out to Oregon?

All of this indexing of possibilities flipped through my mind in the seconds it took him to answer me. "Jean, I am sorry to tell you this, but Ted has cancer. He came to see if he chipped the bone on his shin when he hit it while chopping ice. The X-rays showed a large lesion almost through the large bone of his left leg. I called him back in for a complete nuclear scan today, and it showed a massive tumor on his left kidney, suspicious spots on his lung, ribs and shoulder bones." I could tell he was reading the diagnosis from a paper. All the blood seemed to drain out of my body. I felt numb, cold, empty.

Realizing that Mother lay two feet away, listening, searching my face for clues to what this could be, I calmly replied, "What is the prognosis? I want the truth—absolutely no games!"

He said, "Are you alone?"

I replied quietly, "There is nothing you can't tell me. I will be all right. Just don't pretend or lie to me."

He went on, "The kidney should come out within twenty-four to thirty-six hours. Ted told me of your problems with your mother's illness. I hate to pile this on top, but Ted needs you."

I asked again for an honest answer. Did we have anything to hope with?

"Jean, there really is no hope I can offer you. The leg lesion is a metastasis from the kidney tumor. Once it has spread from the original site, you can try to slow it down with radiation and surgery, but quite honestly, there isn't much anyone can do to really stop it."

I asked, "How much time?"

His voice quietly, but matter-of-factly said, "He might not make it through the surgery. There is really no way of knowing. We are just guessing until we get inside and see the involvement."

I asked how Ted took the news. He said, "Jean, it was the hardest diagnosis I ever reported to a patient. I left the room and came back three times before I could tell him. You and Ted are my friends, as well as my patients. You have such a happy home, nice children—I hated to be the one to tell you it was coming to an end. When I came back in the room the third time, Ted was smiling and said, 'It's O.K., Doc. I read my file when you were out this time. I know the problem. Where do we go from here?' "

Our small, uncomprehending, finite minds had no ruler to measure the depths of anguish, width of despair, or height of pain we had ahead of us. But by the same token, we also had no comprehension of the depth of God's grace, the width of His sufficiency to meet every day we came to, or the height of His continuing strength—His power—His courage—His joy in one of the very darkest, unimaginable, despairing experiences a human being is called upon to go through in life.

Several years before, I had read: "The measure of a man is how he meets disappointment." As I hung up the phone that April morning, I leaned back in the chair and tried to collect myself and arrange my thoughts to meet the challenge of what lay ahead; not only for me, a wife, mother, and daughter—but for all those whose lives would be touched and affected by the news that I had just heard.

First and foremost was Ted. Oh, my dearest! My mind again hurled itself across the frozen miles that separated us. I looked out the window. The sun was still shining. The same little brown bird that I had pointed out to Mother as I bathed her was still darting in and out of the bush outside her window. The same sunshine was streaming in on the carpet as I sat wiggling my toes in its warmth. I felt so cold; I wondered if I would ever feel really warm again. I felt as though my blood had frozen to crystals, and I would crack if I moved too quickly. My eyes saw the same sights and movements—my ears heard the same sounds of living—but I thought, "How different it all looks and sounds and feels than it did before I answered the phone!"

Before I could deal with the long-range problems, I had to face the immediate problem of my extremely ill mother, who, although not knowing exactly what, knew that something major was happening.

After a year of pain, she had undergone major surgery two weeks earlier. I had arrived ten days before to care for her, and was shocked to find her dwarfed among the blankets on the hospital bed; a shrunken tired little lady. She had lost over thirty pounds, and the suffering of the past year was etched on her dear face. About a month before this surgery, Floriene, her constantly faithful friend, had led her gently back to Jesus. I had prayed for her every day of the thirty years that she had bitterly refused God in her life, and I must confess I was surprised when God answered those prayers. How grateful I was that He had!

During the ten days I had been with her, we had achieved a new closeness as we shared our morning and evening devotions. I slept beside her bed on a davenport, and many nights we talked for hours when I could tell from her breathing she was not able to sleep. I tried to encourage her to commit this terrible situation she was in completely to the Lord. I realized that it was easier to be the "sayer" than the "doer," but in her extreme circumstances, I could offer no other help.

I stood on wooden legs and walked to her bedside and took her hand in mine. Tears were streaming down her tired, sick face. Wishing I could think of a believable lie that would spare her and protect her, I had no choice but to tell her the truth. There was no way over it, under it, or around it. We could only go right through the middle of it, by God's Grace.

When I found my voice, it sounded unfamiliar to my ears. "Mother, I wish with all my heart that I didn't have to tell you this. That was Dr. Larson. I must go home today. Ted needs me. He has cancer. Dr. Larson says he should have surgery immediately, but he will wait till I get there. I hate to leave you when you are so sick. I know you need me, but Ted needs me more."

She was speechless. We only pressed each other's hand tightly, and our tears mingled as I leaned over and pressed my face against hers while we tried to comfort each other. She finally said, "Of course you must go. I will be all right. The Lord will just have to take over."

As we clutched each other's hands tightly, I prayed quickly and simply. "Loving Father, we need You! We are Your children, we belong to You. We have given our whole lives to You and prayed for Your guidance in them. We are utterly helpless today—we can only give You this whole horrible situation. We cannot understand why You have allowed this to come into our lives, but we trust You. I'm not asking You to go before us—I'm asking You to stay beside us—in us, around us. Most of all, may others see Jesus Christ in our lives as we face whatever lies ahead."

With this, I walked to the phone. My first priority was getting back to Ted!

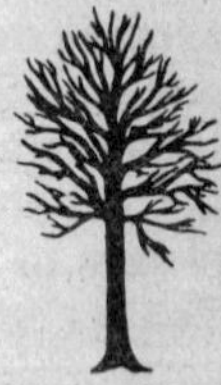

2

It Can't Be True

I had no idea which airlines flew to North Dakota. I simply called Portland International Airport and said, "Connect me with the airline with the first flight to Minot, North Dakota." As she was looking up schedules, my mind raced ahead. I had to call Lorie and get him started home. I had to find a way to the airport. I needed cash for the plane fare.

The operator connected me with North Central. I told the lady I needed a flight out immediately. She said, "I am sorry, but there is no way I can get you out of Portland until tomorrow, at the earliest."

I replied, "I just received a phone call from my doctor. My husband is very ill, he needs me, and I am going on *some* plane today. I don't care if I have to stand in the aisle all the way. I will give you my phone number—you find me a plane. Just tell me what gate and what time, and I will be there!"

I called our son's college and talked to the Boys' Dean. I explained the situation, saying that I wanted Lorie taken out of class and started home. I didn't want him to know the details, as he had a long trip ahead of him alone. I asked the dean to just tell him his dad was sick and we needed him. After a half dozen calls, I finally found Myra. She had been my dearest friend the first years of our marriage, and even though we seldom saw each other since they moved to Oregon, we stayed best friends. She was the kind of friend you find very seldom. I quickly outlined the situation and asked her to take me to the airport by way of the bank.

As I was hurriedly throwing clothes into my suitcases, the airline called with my flight number and estimated time of arrival. With this information, I dialed my home number with fingers that were shaking so badly I could barely make them go around the circle. My stomach still felt like I had been kicked.

Ted answered, and for a few seconds I couldn't make any words come out of my mouth. Oh, the dearness of his voice! How could it be true that the sound of it might soon be stilled? *Surely it couldn't be true!*

After swallowing several times, my voice shaking, I managed to push the words past the massive lump in my throat. "Darling, Dr. Larson just called me. Will you meet me in Bismarck tonight at 10:15?"

"Can you make it that soon?" he said.

"You just be there, sweetheart—I will be on that plane!"

The wires were silent as we both fought for control. He finally said quietly, "I'm glad you are coming, honey. I need you. I love you."

My voice broke as I said, "Hang on. I'll be there!" We

hung up, not daring to say more.

It was very difficult to say goodbye to Mother. She was so terribly sick, and had been depending on me to stay with her through her ordeal. I hated to leave her in such a helpless condition. I thought of the talks and times of prayer that we had shared in the past ten days, and remembered that I had told her over and over that God was sufficient for the very hardest things that life could hand us. There was nothing that He could not and would not give us strength and grace to bear—*if we let Him.*

Several years before, I had found a book by Eugenia Price called *Woman to Woman.* It had revolutionized my life, and I had shared many copies with other women. The main theme of the book was total commitment in *every* phase of our lives. God isn't interested in only our "weekend lives"—He wants total commitment of ourselves, our personalities, our words, our wants, our dislikes, our children, our husbands, our neighbors—everything. Nothing may remain hidden in the closets of our minds—no little hurts to be nursed in secret, no disappointments to be cherished and taken out in the dark of night to be fondled like a rosary, polishing it with our gigantic supply of self-pity.

It was a different situation than standing over her bed and telling her "to do" and "feel" and "be" all of these things—to *let* the Lord be sufficient for her needs. Now I was the one who had to *let* Him prove, in my life, all of the things I had been talking about. I took her hand in both of mine, and as I bent to kiss her goodbye, I said softly, "Mother, I know that you love me, and when someone we love hurts, we hurt too. I want you to commit me to Jesus Christ, just as I have you. Continue to love me and pray for me, but try not to worry about me. I will be all right, I promise you. I will prove to you that God's promises are true!"

I am confident that my feelings that first day are not unusual for the circumstances. Anyone receiving similar news has felt similar emotions of unreality, disbelief, shock, numbness, despair, and fear.

Myra and I had only minutes to spare by the time we found the correct gate, had the luggage checked, and bought my ticket. With a hug, I thanked Myra for driving me to the airport, then hurried to catch my flight.

The plane rose above Portland International Airport, into a sea of white cotton batting. I thought, as I watched the ground fall away from under me: These massive, complex buildings, freeways, and mountains all loom so enormous when we are down in the midst of them, but recede into tiny specks of nothingness as our perspective changes. Could Ted's illness be unimportant and insignificant in God's sight—viewed from His perspective? Could this be a terrible dream, that I would waken from soon? I would go get a drink of water to wake up fully, then go back to bed and crawl over into the circle of Ted's arms and shudder as I was thankful it was only a dream.

I found myself praying constantly—a plea for strength, for courage, for wisdom to know how to face the tumult ahead—for Ted and myself. I tried to plan all of the loving, wise things which would comfort Ted. When you know your time together, barring a miracle, will be limited, what *do* you say?

It was dark when the plane descended into the blaze of lights that was Bismarck, North Dakota. My eyes searched the crowd for Ted's figure. I finally singled him out, standing off to one side alone, his hands deep in his pockets in the biting wind. I was literally shaking from tension, shock, emotions, and cold. I could see him before he could see me, as he was inside the circle of lights from the waiting room. His face was drawn and weary as he searched the crowd getting off the plane.

When I started down the steps, he ran over to the plane, up the last two or three steps, and put his arm around me. When we got to the ground, neither of us could speak at first. We just looked at each other for a long minute, then he wordlessly folded me in his arms. I was going to try to be brave and not cry, but I needn't have bothered, because we both had tears streaming down our cheeks.

At first I couldn't push any words past the lump in my

throat, but I finally managed to say, "Oh, darling, all the long five hours on the plane I planned and prayed for the right comforting words to say to you, and all I can think of now is 'I love you.' "

He smiled, squeezing me till I thought my ribs would crack, and said reassuringly, "Honey, I've never doubted that from the first day I met you."

We clung tightly to each other's hand as we went inside to get my luggage. We didn't trust ourselves to talk in the middle of the hurrying crowd that swirled around us. We tried to look at each other, but that brought tears to our eyes. We didn't dare start with the tears, or there would be no stopping them, so we just hung on tightly to each other's hand and waited until we got out to the car.

After he had helped me in, Ted went around to the driver's side and got in. Immediately, we fell into each other's arms and both wept unashamedly.

When I could finally push some words out, I pulled back in his arms, looked in his eyes, and said, "It simply cannot be true!"

He replied sadly, "I know it. I have felt all day that this is a horrible dream. It could happen to someone else, but not *me!* I've never been sick in my life. I planned to live to be an old man with a white beard, like my grandfather.

"I've worked so hard all my life to be able to retire and take it easy and enjoy our later years. I wanted to travel, to be able to sleep late, to see and do things, and I wanted to share these years with you. How can it be true that I could die—and all of our dreams and plans die with me? It just can't be true! Surely God wouldn't let this happen to me.

"Honey," Ted said, "we will just have to do all we can to get this problem solved. I have faith that God can heal me if it is His will. We will do whatever the doctor says and trust the rest to God. From there on, we will just have to be thankful for the happy years we have had together, and not feel sorry for those we may not get to share."

All at once the realization of what it would mean to be without the security of his presence made me cry, "But I don't want you to die! I love you and need you. The kids need you, the church needs you. I planned to die first. I don't want to be left alone. I don't know how to run a big farm. Why can't it be me?"

He simply held me tighter and assured me of God's plan for our lives and our commitment to Him, reminding me that even without him, I would never be really alone.

It was too bitterly cold to be sitting in a car, so we started home. While Ted drove slowly with one hand, his other arm holding me close, we tried to sort out our thoughts and plans for the next couple of days. The children had to be told, also his parents, our friends, our brothers and sisters. I told Ted that Lorie was on his way home from college and should be there soon. He assured me that he hadn't mentioned anything to Jody. He had simply told her that I was coming home that night. She was to go to bed and could expect us about midnight. I asked if she was suspicious at my coming by plane, and so soon, but he said she didn't question him.

It was a two-hour drive through a moonless, empty night, but we had much to sort out and discuss as he headed for the home we had built, where we had planned to live out our lives together. When we drove up in our yard and I walked into the house, I realized how terrifying the future looked without Ted in it. For a moment it was almost more than I could bear. Without words, he knew how I was feeling, and he took me in his arms and held me close. We didn't trust ourselves to speak.

3

Where Do We Go From Here?

When Jody heard us come in, she greeted us with hugs. We talked briefly about Grandma and about Jody's schoolwork. It wasn't long before the back door burst open and Lorie came bounding in, breathlessly demanding, "Where's Dad? What's wrong?"

Ted came out of the bedroom, and after hugs all around, we sat down together around the table. As we looked at each other, I thought of the many nights we had sat there together, the many meals and happy times we had shared.

Ted and I looked at each other, and his eyes filled with tears. He pressed my hand tightly and said, "You tell them. I can't!"

I closed my eyes and begged, "Oh, heavenly Father, *help me!*" I told them as quickly and simply as I could. There is no easy or kind way to tell children that their father has cancer. It was simply a fact that had to be faced.

I explained first that we had never lied to them because we didn't want them to lie to us. Our first thought was to protect them; to make life easy and fun for them. Pretending it wasn't so, would not make it disappear.

Of course they were stunned, as we had been hours before. Jody said that she was suspicious when the nurse called Ted to come back to the office for more tests. She imagined it might be serious, but not *that* serious!

The four of us sat, numb and hardly believing the truth, as we had our family devotions. Then we held hands for prayer. Of course tears could not be held back, and I prayed simply, quietly, and from my heart.

"Loving Father, we are Thy children. We belong to You, we love You. We do not understand why You have allowed this trial to come into our lives. We can only trust that You have a plan for us. The coming days will be difficult, long, and frightening—be our strength, give us Your courage, Your peace.

"Tonight we are confused, frightened, and just plain scared. Help us to hang on tightly to Your hand and give us confidence that You will hold tightly to *us*. We really don't know how or what to pray, only that You heal Daddy, if it is Your will. We need him, we love him. Please don't take him away from us! Most of all, we love Thee. Help us, that others will see Jesus Christ shining through our lives in the difficult days ahead. We commit our lives totally to You again tonight. Be in us, shine through us, use us, but most of all, *help us!*"

Jody came and hugged and kissed both of us through her tears, then went wordlessly to her room. Lorie kissed me and started to shake hands with Ted, but then they hugged each other without words before he went to his room.

I went into Jody's room and sat on her bed. Taking her hand, I asked if she was all right and did she want me to lie down beside her for a little while. She said, "No, Mother, I'll be all right. You stay with Daddy—he needs you the most tonight."

As Ted and I silently prepared for bed, it seemed that my body was not mine; that I was sitting off in a corner watching me—watching another woman. She looked like me, tired from the trip, tense and concerned from the stress of the situation. But the me in the corner couldn't feel what the real me felt as I got my nightgown out of the drawer, took off my shoes, and pulled down the bedspread. She seemed without substance or reality. Her legs and arms felt as if they were made of plastic. She was moving mechanically, more like a robot than a real person.

Whenever I returned home from visiting my folks, Ted always had a note on my pillow. Often containing some silliness, it would also hold something warm and dear. We were great note senders. I usually sent a note in his lunch if he went someplace to work, or in his pocket if he went away for the day to a meeting. No great words of wisdom, but just to assure him that I loved him and was anxious for him to come home to me at the day's end. For all of the twenty-two years of our marriage, whenever I came home from a trip, he had not failed to have a note waiting for me.

This night I was surprised to find that he had gone ahead with this tradition. I thought "Oh, how can he think of our foolish nonsense at such a serious time?" I opened the short note, fearing what I would read. "Welcome home again, darling—to our home, to my heart, to my arms. Thank you for coming so quickly. I need you. I love you, with all my heart, for all of my life." I couldn't even cry. I just felt dazed, numb, hovering on the edge of a desolate abyss, and more tired than I had ever felt before in my life.

It was almost 2 A.M. as I lay down woodenly on the soft,

cool, clean sheets. Ted was sitting on Jody's bed, talking to her, assuring her that we would find a way through the situation and do our best.

At last he came into the bedroom and undressed without saying anything or even looking at me. I watched him as he did all the dear, familiar things; putting his change and his wallet on the dresser, emptying his pockets, getting out clean sox and underwear for the morning, hanging up his slacks. I watched him, still dry-eyed, amazed I could look at him and even consider this might be coming to an end for us. *How? Why?—It simply could not be true!*

We really loved each other. So many couples simply put up with each other or else lead lives of quiet (or not-so-quiet) desperation. Why, when we were so happy? Why couldn't someone else die, who wasn't happy or didn't want to live? Oh, please God—don't let this be true!

Switching off the light, Ted lay down with a big sigh of weariness. For half a minute he remained motionless, then turning, he drew me close, and again we cried together. There just weren't any new words—we had said all of them before.

What new words could we find? Only the same ones, over and over again. I could only say, "Why? . . .

"It can't be true!

"I need you, the children need you.

"What will I do?"

From Ted: "I don't want to die—there must be some other way. Surely God will heal me. I am busy working for Him.

"I have never done anything really bad in my whole life.

"Surely I am worth more to Him alive than dead!"

Our misery was compounded by our need to find a way of escape from this black, horrible painful monster that had invaded our lives.

Suddenly I thought of Lorie. We had known this for a day, but he just learned of it an hour ago. What a frightening experience this must be for him. I suggested that Ted go down and talk to Lorie, so he got up, put on his robe and slippers, and went downstairs.

When he came back a half hour later, he couldn't talk for a few minutes. He finally said, "I thought my heart would break. I found this big six-foot-two nineteen-year-old with his head under the covers, sobbing. I sat down beside him and put my arms around him and we cried together.

"Lorie wanted to know *why,* and I didn't have any answers. What could I say? I don't know the reason for *me*—how can I give him a reason for *him?* I told him that he had to be brave, that we would make it, somehow. It was a lot to dump in a teenager's lap, but I had confidence that he could do it. He would have to grow up fast and be the man of the family. I said I had confidence in him and knew that he could do it."

We spent the rest of the night sleeplessly, simply holding each other closely and talking quietly of what to do first. *Where do we go from here?*

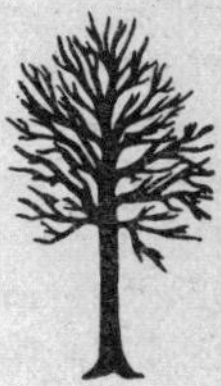

4

Journey Through the Valley

The next day we went into Minot to make arrangements for the hospitalization and surgery. Dr. Larson had encouraged Ted to see a lawyer and make out a will before he was admitted to the hospital, so he did that in town, too. Ted's next youngest brother, Ed, was a minister. I had called Ed's wife from the airport in Spokane during a stopover on the way home and asked them to come be with us that next day. They met us at the hospital and returned home with us.

In talking it over on the way home, we decided that Ted should go to the Mayo Clinic, in Rochester, Minnesota. We felt that at Mayo, Ted would get the very best medical help in the world. Dr. Larson phoned ahead to cut through the red tape and made an appointment for the next day.

Ted's youngest brother, Jim, was a pilot, so he and his wife, Diane, flew us to Rochester the next morning. Although Dr. Larson had given us the forty-eight X-rays that were taken in Minot, Mayo did a complete workup, and their diagnosis was the same: "Renal carcinoma, metastasis to the left tibia, possible involvement of the ribs, shoulder, lung." Surgery was scheduled for the following Tuesday morning.

Meanwhile, ahead of us stretched a long weekend. We had no car, since we had flown down, and walking was painful for Ted. The days were long and anxious, knowing the children were alone, and loved ones concerned. However, we were soon to see God's love and care manifest itself in an unusual way.

I had noticed a small sign beside the elevator at the clinic, saying there was a room in the annex of a small church across the street where there were books, toys for children, cookies and punch, even people with whom to visit between appointments. After we had eaten, we walked over there and met the world's friendliest man, Ed Burfiend. In talking together, we discovered he was a retired farmer, now a sexton at the church during the day and a maintenance man at the clinic from 5:30 P.M. to 2:30 A.M. Despite his busy schedule, he appeared to have boundless energy. The man must have had helium in his blood! He could work endless hours and seem to work just as hard at the end as at the beginning, then bounce right back, ready to go the next day.

He called his wife, Marie, and they invited us out for the evening. The Lord certainly was preparing a special place for us. Before the evening was over, they had invited us to move into their guest room. They had no children, both worked, so the house was to be ours most of the time. We had no hospitalization insurance, and to have to live in a hotel, eating in a restaurant for two or three months, would have been horribly expensive. Here again was a definite expression of God's loving, watchful care over us. Ed and Marie became our dear, kind friends in the days ahead. Ed dropped me off at the hospital at 7:00 A.M. on his way to work each morning, and Marie came and picked me up at 10:00 each night.

The weekend seemed endless. Although we treasured each moment we had to share, it was a long, frightening couple of days. Bill and Margaret—our dear friends who were the first I had called with the news of Ted's illness—were in Minneapolis, visiting her sister and brother-in-law, so they drove down for dinner with us Sunday afternoon. Afterward, we visited in a little park for an hour or two. When they finally had to leave, they wanted to take us back to the hotel, but Ted said it was only about four blocks, and he wanted to walk.

After saying tearful goodbyes to our friends, we started walking back, holding hands, not talking, just sharing the closeness of being together. Passing a baseball game between college-age fellows, Ted slowed down until he stood pressed against the fence, listening to the good-natured bickering and yells "for" and boos "against." I saw, mirrored in the pain on Ted's face, memories of his love of playing ball and the stark realization that he would no doubt never play again. With Ted clutching my hand still tighter, we resumed our journey.

He was exhausted when we got back to our hotel room, and lay down on the bed, asking me to read to him. In our book of devotions, *Streams in the Desert* by Mrs. Charles Cowman, I came upon a couple of paragraphs which were to sustain not only us, but many of our friends in the weeks and months ahead. Ted lay quietly with his eyes shut, holding on to my hand as I read:

> *"Consider the work of God: for who can make that straight, which he hath made crooked." (Ecclesiastes 7:13.)*
>
> Often God seems to place His children in positions of profound difficulty, leading them into a wedge from which there is no escape; contriving a situation which no human judgment would have permitted, had it been previously consulted . . . . *You may be thus involved at this very hour.*

It does seem perplexing and very serious to the last degree, but it is perfectly right. The issue will more than justify Him who has brought you hither. *It is a platform for the display of His almighty grace and power.*

It puzzles me; but, Lord, Thou understandest,
And wilt one day explain this crooked thing.
Meanwhile, I know that it has worked out Thy best—
Its very crookedness taught me to cling.
Thou hast fenced up my ways, made my paths crooked,
To keep my wand'ring eyes fixed on Thee,
To make me what I was not, humble, patient;
To draw my heart from earthly love to Thee.
So I will thank and praise Thee for this puzzle,
And trust where I cannot understand.
Rejoicing Thou dost hold me worth such testing.
I cling the closer to Thy guiding hand.
—F.E.M.I.

Tears were streaming down both of our faces by the time I was through. Kneeling beside that hotel bed, we again committed our lives—to live or die—to Jesus Christ. We knew that, in ourselves, we had no strength for the weeks ahead. Anything we could be or do would have to be by His strength. Earnestly we prayed that He would use our lives as a *platform for the display of His almighty grace and power.* The future looked frightening, vast, dark, and unknown, but we trusted Him to use our lives and this seeming tragedy to *prove* God's promises are true!

Ted entered St. Mary's Hospital the next day, scheduled for surgery to remove his kidney the following morning. I stayed with him until they gave him a sedative for the night's rest, and was back at the hospital at 6:00 A.M. the next morning. When the nurse came in to get him ready, she was careful to avoid all mention of his surgery, but she needn't have bothered. Ted was his usual, cheery self.

Before leaving the room. we committed Ted's life to

Jesus Christ. We were not afraid. We didn't know what the next few hours would mean in terms of life or death, but we were confident that we belonged to Him, and He would see us through.

By 7:00 A.M., I was walking down the corridor beside the gurney, holding Ted's hand. When we got to the elevator, I hugged him, sending him off with kisses and smiles, confident he would be back soon.

I returned to his room to collect my Bible, book of devotions, and stationery before going to the waiting room. I later received many letters expressing concern that I was so far from home and had to go through that day by myself. Not once in all those many long hours of waiting and praying did I ever feel alone! Instead, I felt completely surrounded by God's loving, warm, sheltering arms.

In the waiting room, I heard a man across from me sharing with a woman sitting nearby that his wife was in surgery for breast cancer. As he chain-smoked and walked the floor anxiously, rambling on about his fear and pain, my heart ached for those who must go through any tragedy without the strengthening power of God's love.

I read. I prayed. I wrote letters to our parents and the children. Still no word came from surgery about Ted. His operation had been scheduled for seven-thirty. The nurse told me later that the patients are lined up in long rows and taken one by one. There was a little girl, with a large tumor on her head, who lay frightened and crying. Ted asked the doctor to give her his place in the schedule. That was so typical of Ted that I wasn't surprised when she told me.

About noon, a doctor came and told the man whose wife was in surgery that they had waited too long; there was nothing they could do. Due to complications, his wife would probably not live through the day. He just sat there after the doctor left, stunned, not knowing where to go or what to do.

I went over and asked if he would like a drink of water or if there was someone I could call for him. Slowly raising eyes that were swimming in tears, he whispered, "What will I do? I have no one, besides me, who will even care.

What will I do? What will I do?"

I brought him a drink of water and he finally got shakily to his feet and wandered aimlessly down the hall—a picture of utter hopelessness and fear.

Again I thanked the Lord for His presence there with me. I did not feel any fear or sense of hopelessness. I felt completely cushioned and upheld by God's loving arms. This feeling of warmth and trust did not fade as the hours got longer and longer, and still no word came about Ted.

I knew that it would be a long, involved surgery, and didn't expect him back for several hours. But when the wait went to four and five hours, I couldn't help but wonder what was taking so long.

Finally, after seven hours, a nurse came and asked me to follow her. One of the surgeons wanted to speak to me in pathology. I quickly asked if she had any word if Ted was still alive or not, and she replied, "No, the only message that came down was that you were to go upstairs so the doctor could talk to you."

I must confess that this was a frightening turn of events. I closed my eyes and pleaded for His strength and courage to face whatever the next few moments held for me.

My fears were intensified a few minutes later, when I got upstairs to the surgery floor, and right outside the door of the pathology department stood an *empty* gurney. My instant reaction was that Ted must have died and they brought me up here to tell me what had happened, rather than downstairs in front of people!

Happily, I was wrong.

The doctor introduced himself and assured me that Ted was still alive, but added that their fears about the involvement were not groundless. He asked me if he could show me what they had removed from Ted. I thought to myself, "Now being brave is one thing, but can I honestly face this bloody mass that was a part of Ted until just a few minutes ago?"

I was not squeamish about fixing cuts, bloody noses, and the usual problems that are part of raising children, but really questioned my ability to face this. There was no time to psych myself up or steel myself. I managed to mumble yes from between wooden lips, and he set a tray in front of me and removed the white napkin.

On the tray lay a large, white, porous, spongy-looking mass. The smaller, reddish-brown, bean-shaped object, he explained, was Ted's kidney. Only about two inches of the kidney stuck out from the porous mass; the rest was completely enveloped by it. The mass had been cut in two. Opening it up, the doctor showed me how it had started within the kidney, finally growing outside, completely enveloping it.

I sat stunned and disbelieving as I looked at the offending foreign monster which had invaded Ted's body, changing our lives. Where had it come from? What would its ultimate effect be on our lives? Again—*why?* I stared at it wordlessly, while the doctor's voice droned on and on about the technical reasons, what they had found, what they had done, and what we could expect.

My main concern was for Ted's immediate condition and safety. Finishing the technical explanations, the doctor asked if I had any questions. Raising my eyes from the tray, I replied, "Only one thing I care about: What does this mean to Ted's present condition? Do we have any kind of hope for the future?"

He hesitated before answering. "Mrs. Scheresky," he said, clearing his throat, "at Mayo Clinic we try to have the best doctors, equipment, and diagnostic services available. We try not to take the patient's hope away. But since you asked for the complete truth, there really is no hope for Mr. Scheresky's recovery, other than a miracle. We cannot tell where the cancer came from, or what caused it, but once it has metastasized—moved to another site—it will continue to spread. It is simply a matter of time.

"The kidney," he said, "is a filter for the blood for the whole body, and these cancer cells have spread all over his body. We have removed the original site, and depending on his ability to survive this massive surgery today, we will go in, as soon as he is able, and try to cope with the leg lesion. Then we will just wait to see where it will surface on another part of his body. If it has invaded one lung, we can use radiation therapy to slow it down, and even remove one lung; but when it spreads to the other one, there isn't anything we can do. We will simply watch and wait and deal with whatever appears, when it appears.

"Mr. Scheresky's surgery this morning was very involved," he said. "That is why it took so long. We estimate that the tumor has been growing for at least two or three years, and the many complications made the surgery an extremely difficult task. He survived the surgery partly because he was such a strong, healthy man to begin with, and he has a tremendous will to survive. After we got him under the anesthetic, the operating-room crew remarked what an unusual fellow he must be. He had been laughing and trying to cheer up everyone around him. His last remark before he was unconscious was, 'Doc, I don't care how deep you go, or what you cut out, just so you get me back downstairs to my wife and kids. Don't be nervous or worried about me. I know I'm going to be all right. You do your part, and God will do mine.' "

Those first three days following surgery were a jumbled, hazy dream to Ted. The fourth day, he was out of bed and shuffling to the door and back. By the end of the sixth day, he was making a very slow trip to the end of the hall and back, supported by two nurses, a third one pulling the suction machine still attached to the incision on his back. His "railroad tracks," as he called his incision, curved from up near his shoulder blade, down under the arm, and around to the front of his side. The suction machine was finally removed the morning before he was taken back to surgery for his leg.

Two orthopedic specialists wanted to remove the offending leg at the thigh, but Ted begged them not to. If at all possible, could they please try to save it? They couldn't promise, so he went to surgery not knowing if he would come back with or without his leg.

Surgery was scheduled for 11:00 A.M. By 6:30 in the evening, he hadn't come back. Even the nurses were worried enough to call upstairs a couple of times to see if he was all right. Finally, at 7:00, one of the student nurses came flying down from the station.

"They just called to get Scheresky's bed ready with hot

water bottles. He's in shock, but they are bringing him down!"

The hall was lined with all the nurses, aides, and student nurses. One was peeking around the corner to the elevator, and she suddenly whirled around and shouted, "Here he comes, and he's got two legs!" All the nurses cheered, and mine were not the only cheeks wet with tears.

This time, he was not so spunky when he came out of the anesthetic. He was in a great deal of pain, because the doctors had taken out six inches of bone from the main shinbone. They made an incision on his knee and pounded a steel rod down through the bone marrow from his knee to his ankle, filled in the six inches of missing bone with plastic cement around the steel rod, and sewed it up. Finally, the leg was encased in a steel cast. Ted commented later that this surgery was ten times more painful than the kidney.

The following weeks were the most painful of all, but Ted never complained. The medication made him hallucinate when awake and have terrible nightmares when he slept, so he finally just refused it. He preferred pain to the nightmares. He was so very grateful that he hadn't lost his leg, and remained confident he was "going to beat this thing" and God was going to heal him.

He was anxious to get to physical therapy and learn to walk again with crutches. He begged the doctor to let him try it, so it was with great excitement and anticipation that we were finally given permission for me to take him down to physical therapy.

He fainted from pain that first day, but went back the next day, determined to be mobile again; which of course he was, little by little.

After three weeks, Ted was released from the hospital to the outpatient clinic, thirty-two pounds lighter and very weak. He still had to report every morning for radiation therapy, but he could be "home" the rest of the time.

It was a very happy man that I took home from the hospital that day, I assure you. When I rolled the wheelchair outside, he begged me to stop and pull a handful of grass from the lawn. Burying his nose in it, he declared that it was better than any perfume he'd ever smelled.

We were full of hope and confidence. The three more weeks we had to stay in Rochester for radiation treatments were full of gratefulness and praise that we'd made it this far. We were confident God would see us through the rest of the way.

We had called the children every day. They were only fifteen and nineteen, and this was a frightening experience for them. We wanted to share with them our concern and support, and assure them how proud we were of them for keeping things going at home.

When it was time for us to go home and let Ted try to get some strength back, Jim flew down to get us and our son, Lorie, came with him. I can't tell you how good that long-legged boy that came running across the airfield looked to us.

Jody was at the airfield in Minot to meet our plane, and it was a happy family that gathered around our table that night for dinner. Our hearts were full of joy that the Lord had let us be together again.

Time for spring's work had arrived while we were gone, and we both shed tears of gratefulness after receiving a card and letter telling us of the neighbors who had come and put in our crops for us. The card was signed by each of the men and by the ladies who had provided the food and cooked the meals. When we returned home, I put the following in the newspaper:

> Two little words—"thank you"—seem so inadequate to express our appreciation to our family, friends, and neighbors for the cards, calls and letters of loving concern the weeks Ted has been in the hospital in Rochester. Our special appreciation to the twenty-eight neighbors who left their own delayed spring's work, to come and do ours. Thank you from the bottom of our hearts. Do not fear for us, we are totally committed to Jesus Christ. If this is the path He has chosen for us, we are willing to walk in it.
>
> The Ted Scheresky Family

5

You Are the Sunshine of My Life

The next month was a *busy* one. Spring had come and gone quickly in the northern prairies. Jody had kept the lawn mowed, but nothing had been done to all of the flower beds, and they looked like a jungle. There was a big garden to be put in and tended. Summer on the farm is a busy time.

Ted was so thrilled to be home. He was discouraged that his strength did not match his ambition. He and Jim had ordered a new tractor before he got sick, and he had never ridden it. I begged him to be patient and wait a while before trying it out, but Lorie confided to me that his dad couldn't resist the temptation, and he did make one round with him, but he didn't quibble about getting off. It was too rough for him so soon after such big operations. It was so difficult for him to have to lie down every couple of hours when there was so much work to be done. He was not the lie-down-and-be-sick type.

The first weekend home, he could hardly wait to go to church. Oh, it was so good to be back among friends who we knew loved us and had been praying for us. Shakily, Ted went up on the platform of our little country church. As he put his crutches under his chair and stood to lead in prayer, his voice broke as he thanked God for sparing him and bringing us all together again.

The month sped by, and soon we had to return to Rochester for another full month of radiation treatments. July was hot and muggy, but we were happy to be getting help and were still confident with the hope the doctors had given us that he could "beat it"; at least for a couple of years. We had done as the Bible admonished us, we had called for the elders of the church and prayed for him. Surely God would hear us, and answer as we had asked. Ted had been serving the Lord all his life. *Surely* the Lord would heal him, or at least grant him another year of so—wouldn't He . . . ?

Ted's doctor was out of town over a long weekend. It was a very hot, humid day, and the power was down, so the air conditioner was not working. Ted decided to take a cool bath. When he took his elastic sock off his bad leg we were shocked to see it terribly swollen. He said, "You better call the doctor. I don't know what that could mean!"

The doctor who was on call knew nothing of Ted's case. He simply looked up his chart and stated matter-of-factly, "Oh, that must mean the tumor is growing fast again."

An icy hand clutched my heart, and I could scarcely find the breath to reply. "We were told that they had removed the tumor, and the radiation was to take care of any residual cells."

"Lady," he said tiredly, "I'm reading his diagnosis from his chart. I don't know what they told you, but your husband is going to die, and you better get used to the idea."

Ted was lying on the davenport not ten feet away, watching me. I couldn't think of what to say. I couldn't tell my brave, trusting, confident husband he was going to die! I couldn't make any words come out at all. Finally, I simply and quietly hung up the phone on the puzzled doctor's still-talking voice.

I numbly helped Ted into the bathroom and ran a tepid bath for him. He went on talking about the heat, but I was mute in the face of the vast and dark unknown stretching out ahead of me. I think my hope started to die a little that day.

The next month was one of the most difficult for me. Before, we had faced everything together. When we were told he was going to die, we cried together and prayed together. All through the long, dark, painful days and weeks of the surgeries and recoveries, we hoped and had faith together. That next month, when he still had great faith and high hopes (but I could see him going downhill, as the doctor had told me he would), was the hardest time. Not sharing my grief and pain with him was torture.

The radiation treatments finally slid to an end, and the six-hundred-mile trip home was made shorter by our happiness at being with the children again.

As often happens, the last twenty miles seemed the longest. When I drove into our driveway, Ted's dog came bounding out to meet us. I had barely brought the car to a stop before Ted had the door open and Ruff climbed into the car, laid his head in Ted's lap, and looked up at him with such sorrowful, expressive eyes, as if to say: "Where have you been? I thought you were gone forever. Is this really you?" We were both choked with emotion at the wealth and range of feelings expressed by that dear, faithful, black dog that afternoon.

We arrived home the first of August to a garden, yard, and farm screaming for attention.

Ted glowed with happiness to be near the family and friends he loved. He never expressed a word of discouragement or lack of confidence that God was going to work out His best for our lives. Many friends came to visit him, some hesitantly, who told me they didn't know what to say to a man who had cancer. Although painfully thin and weak, Ted was nothing but optimistic about his future.

I was busy outside much of the time, but except for taking a rest often during the day, Ted stayed near me. If I went to the garden to weed, he would come on his crutches, and I would take along a lawn chair. He would enjoy the sunshine and the birds and the ducks in the lake below the garden. We talked freely of our happy years together and how grateful we were that God had given us twenty-two years to share.

One afternoon, after looking out over the lake silently for quite a while, he said, "One of the reasons I hate to die is because I wanted to grow old with you."

"Oh, darling," I teased, "just think, you won't have to get old and wrinkled and bent. You will always be remembered as young and handsome."

He laughed and then, in a more serious tone, said, "Oh, sweetheart, I had so many plans for us to be happy in the next twenty years. I can't bear to think of not sharing them with you."

I kept digging furiously. I didn't dare answer him. That was the summer "You Are the Sunshine of My Life" was played constantly on the radio. Each time it came on, we'd reach out to touch each other, reassuring ourselves that we were still together. Ted really was the sunshine—everything that was bright, warm, good, and shining in my life. I tried not to think about the dark, cold emptiness that would envelop me without him.

One warm summer morning he was sitting in the lawn chair, watching me plant new bulbs along the block-long driveway to the mailbox. Ted made me move the chair along as I worked. He remarked wistfully, "It doesn't seem possible that next year, when these flowers bloom, I won't be here to see them. Please think of me when they bloom. Whenever you walk to the mailbox, know I loved you and wish that I could be here too."

Those were tender, painful times, but I cherish them. As tired as I got physically, the stress of the situation compounding my weariness, I could only search out God's promises and claim each one as my own. I discovered in His Word that everything which comes into our lives can become a means of blessing—or, if we let it, can crush us into misery and despair. Within each of us lies the power to choose.

Still today, after all that we went through, nothing has dimmed my confidence and faith that God *could* have performed a miracle and healed Ted. I do not doubt one iota God's *ability* to heal Ted. We had done all He asked us to do, and simply accepted His answer to us.

We could do nothing else but trust Him, and we did. Not without tears, not without questioning, but still with complete confidence that He had a plan for our lives. Even though it wasn't what we had chosen, we still could trust Him. Those days of waiting were full of quiet confidence that God would work out His very best for us.

The days were filled with joy at being home again. Lorie and Jim were busy with harvest, and Ted rode in the pickup with Lorie whenever he felt he could, so happy to be part of his world again.

Lorie had an old race car that he was working on in the evenings, and Ted stood on his crutches and helped him when he could. He was every child's wish for a loving, concerned father.

Summer is short, but because of the beauty of the mornings, Ted often encouraged me to get up and watch the sunrise with him. Because he slept often during the day, he didn't sleep well at night. It seemed that he didn't want to waste his time sleeping. He would grab a jacket from a hanger by the back door for us to sit on, and with a flourish, offer me a grandstand seat to "watch God's miracle" of another new day. I would sit there barefoot in my nightgown, with his arm around me in the early morning chill, and we would talk until it was time to get the children up and get on with the duties of the day. When he couldn't sleep at night, he would ask me to get up and sit on the back steps and watch the moon's shining reflection in the lake. It was a breathtaking sight. One night, when there was a full moon, he pulled me up off the step and said, "Come on—let's go teeter-totter!" I had to laugh at the thought of us—two middle-aged people, he in his pajamas and me in my summer nightie—teeter-tottering in the moonlight. I said, "Oh, sweetheart—some men give their wives furs and jewels, but I will bet there aren't very many who give their wives memories of teeter-tottering under a full moon on a warm June night! I wouldn't trade them for anything."

Within two weeks of being home, Ted started complaining of severe headaches. When it didn't get any better, we went to see Dr. Larson. He merely asked how Ted was feeling in general and prescribed pain pills. I wanted Ted to rest more, worrying that he was overdoing what strength he had. I wrote to his doctor at the Mayo Clinic, to ask if the ultimate outcome of his illness would be affected by his rest, or lack of it. The doctor replied it would neither hurry nor slow his illness—to let him do anything he felt well enough to do.

My youngest sister, Susie, called me from Washington and shared something that changed my attitude. I was telling her how concerned I was because Ted didn't take it easy enough, considering all he had been through.

"Sissie, I know you love Ted so much you want to protect and preserve him as long as you can, but don't keep him from going outside. He loves the outdoors, and has spent his whole adult life working and building up that farm. It is beautiful, and he loves every clump of dirt and blade of grass on it. This may be his last summer—let him enjoy it. Let him lie in the grass, let him walk in the lake if he wants to. Let him do anything that will bring him joy."

Those wise words really helped me to realize that my worrying about Ted was really selfish. I wanted to keep him near me as long as possible. I was trying to lock him up in a little cage of my concern. While it would have possibly lengthened his life to a small degree, the quality would have suffered. From that day on, *I let him go* to find what gave him happiness and to savor each moment with special love and joy.

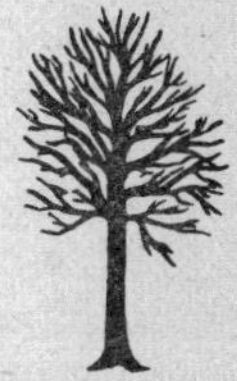

6
It's Just a Matter of Time

As the days passed and he didn't noticeably improve, Ted wondered why the Lord delayed his feeling better. One afternoon he called me to the living room to listen to the following from *Streams in the Desert:*

> When God delays, He is not inactive. He is getting ready His instruments, He is ripening our powers; and at the appointed moment we shall arise equal to our task.
>
> Dr. Jowett
>
> God is never in a hurry but spends years with those He expects to greatly use. He never thinks the days of preparation too long or too dull.
>
> The hardest ingredient in suffering is often *time*. A short, sharp pang is easily borne, but when a sorrow drags its weary way through long, monotonous years, and day after day returns with the same dull routine of hopeless agony, the heart loses its strength, and without the grace of God, is sure to sink into the very sullenness of despair . . . . Don't steal tomorrow out of God's hands. Give God time to speak to you to reveal His will.

When he finished reading to me, Ted said, "Oh, I hope the Lord is patient with me when I am so impatient with Him and His timetable. If God's answer to me is "No," I want to show people nothing but peace and joy in accepting His plan, not mine." I could only numbly and wordlessly nod my head.

I usually slept very lightly, hearing every time Ted turned over; but with the long hours of working outside, I must have been exhausted, because I wakened one night to realize he was getting back into bed. I scooted over to his side to put my arm around him, and he was icy cold.

"Where have you been to get half-frozen?"

"I've been outside. You'd better not come near me. I must have the flu—I'm terribly nauseated, dizzy, and having terrific chills."

All the next day he vomited, the room seemed to revolve constantly, and he had almost unbearable pains in his head. By morning of the second day, he finally conceded that this must be more than the flu, and asked me to call the Minot Air Force Hospital about being admitted. He was far too ill to make the long trip back to the Mayo Clinic.

Within thirty minutes, arrangements were completed and we were on our way. Even with his eyes shut, the light increased the pain in Ted's head, so we kept a folded towel over his eyes. The trip was a nightmare. He didn't know who he was, or who I was, part of the time. I knelt on the floor of the back seat, holding him in my arms, trying to soothe and calm him.

When we arrived at the hospital, the corpsmen lifted Ted into a wheelchair and took us to an examining room to wait for a doctor. We were there only minutes when he lost consciousness. I tried to hold him up, but he was dead weight and slid out of my arms onto the floor. After easing him down gently, I ran into the hall and found a corpsman. Even the two of us couldn't get him back up onto an examining table without the aid of another corpsman.

We didn't wait long before a tall, thin, young doctor came in. Gently smoothing back the hair from Ted's sweaty forehead, he asked, "What's your trouble, Ted? Tell me where you hurt, and I'll do everything I can to help you." We didn't realize at that moment how involved our lives would be with this young man. He was surely another evidence of God's watch-care for us; no one could have been kinder, more gentle, dearer to us both, and more helpful to Ted than this young Air Force captain was.

Captain John Ingram III was to become a trusted and dear friend, as well as Ted's doctor, in the months to come. He told me later that the moment he looked into Ted's eyes with his ophthalmoscope, he could see the pressure on Ted's brain, and knew that the cancer had spread. After admitting him, he immediately started intravenous feeding and Decadron, a steroid medicine. It seemed like magic—within twenty-four hours, most of the symptoms disappeared. Although it doesn't heal anything, Decadron relieves the suffering and is one of the newest drugs for combating cancer. That day, we really thought that the end was near, but by the next morning, the terrible vertigo and pain were both almost gone.

The next two weeks were full of tests of every kind. Dr. Ingram came to see Ted several times each day, and was always encouraging and kind to him. We waited anxiously after the testing was completed, to learn the results and to hear if we had anything else to hope for.

Finally one morning, Dr. Ingram brought another man, a physician's assistant, with him. Ted was sitting up on the edge of his bed. He was feeling so much better, he had great faith they were bringing us good news. Ted smiled and held out his hand to shake hands with both doctors. I felt sorry for Dr. Ingram as I watched his face.

"I'm sorry to have to give you bad news, Ted. The cancer has spread in your lungs. Where there was only one suspicious spot when you were admitted two weeks ago, now there are five. We have not located the exact spot, but we are sure that the cancer has also spread to your brain."

Ted hurriedly broke in and said, "But at Mayo's they said that even if one lung got bad, they could remove it. I can live a long time with one lung. That doesn't mean I won't last a long time yet!"

Dr. Ingram swallowed and looked down at the floor. The other doctor hurriedly said, "We are sorry, Ted, but the new lesions are in your other lung. Now both lungs are involved. That means there isn't anything we can do—it is just a matter of time."

Again, the by-now familiar, red-hot stab in the stomach, and the icy hand on my heart.

Ted bowed his head for a moment, then raised eyes glistening with unshed tears. He again held out his hand to both doctors and thanked them for their kindness, their honesty, and their help. He had asked for the honest truth, he didn't want to play any games, the stakes were too high. They turned and quietly left the room.

I moved quickly to the side of his bed and put my arms around him. We were both stunned. Although we knew this possibility was a very real one, to actually hear the words and know that this was *it,* was a very emotion-filled moment. Neither of us could speak for long, tense moments. We just held each other tightly.

He finally burst out with, "I wish you could just open that window and let me save everyone all the grief and heartache of watching me die!"

I said, "Darling, at this moment I don't blame you for feeling like that. I feel like it would be easier to not only open the window, but take your hand and jump with you! But we really don't have any choice. When this thing started, we told people that if this was the path God had chosen for us, we were willing to walk in it. There are too many people watching our lives. We have no choice but to follow where He leads us. We may not *like* this path; it is rough and stormy, but it is *His* path, and we must follow!"

That one afternoon was the only time, in all of the seven months it took Ted to die, that I saw or heard him discouraged. The rest of the day he lay quietly, and when he asked me to lie down next to him, I did. I am sure Dr. Ingram must have told them at the nurses' station not to bother us, knowing this would be a difficult time for us, for we were only disturbed by the nurse bringing his medicine and the corpsman to take his blood pressure.

I lay on top of the covers with my head on his shoulder, and I think if a nurse had said anything about it, Ted would have not said anything, but he would have gotten up and left the hospital, rather than let me go.

When the corpsman came to take his blood pressure, Ted said, "I may be dying, but you are blind. You *do not* see my wife lying on this bed with my arm around her. You *will not* report it to the head nurse." The corpsman smiled and said, "Ted, I am deaf, dumb, and blind!"

I read to him during most of the evening, since his eyesight had deteriorated badly and he could not read for himself. I hated to leave him that night. I feared he would not sleep, but as I kissed him good-night he said, "Don't worry about me. I will be all right. You were right—I was stunned for a few moments. I had such faith that God was going to heal me. Until this afternoon I still had hope that somehow a miracle might happen, but I am willing to accept God's plan for us.

"I still don't understand, when so many people are watching our lives, *why* He doesn't heal me. Wouldn't that mean more to people if I were healed, than if I die?"

I searched frantically in my mind for something comforting to say. All I could think of was, "Darling, I can't tell you why. The only thing I can think of is that He can use your death more than He can use your life."

At that moment, beside that hospital bed on the sixth floor of the John Moses Air Force Hospital in Minot, North Dakota, I must confess that I did not *really believe* that that could honestly be true. *How* could God use Ted's death? But, looking back over the months that followed, I can see. I do not like it. It was not easy. I wish it were not so. But I can see . . . .

When I left, as I went by the nurses' station, the nurse on duty came and put her arm around me. She said, "I know this has been a terribly difficult day for you. It has been for all of us, too. We have never known a patient like Ted before and I assure you that every nurse on this floor cried when Dr. Ingram told us what he had to tell you today.

"He left orders for a hypo for Ted tonight so he will

sleep, so you go home and don't worry about him. You must get some rest, as he needs you. Don't worry about him tonight, though."

I whispered "Thank you" through my tears as I rode down in the elevator. Again I thanked the Lord for His loving arms and His strength.

As I walked out into the cold, black night to our car, I looked up at Ted's window. He was standing there, watching me. When I blinked the car lights and he waved at me, I thought my heart would break. But it didn't—just another crack in it.

When I arrived the next morning, he was refreshed from his deep sleep of the night, and was his usual happy, smiling, teasing self.

Ted's courage was far greater than mine. He was the one who was facing death: I was just feeling sorry for myself, that I was losing him. Ted finally accepted that his time was definitely limited now, but he still wanted to do all he could to live. He hoped for another six months, at least.

Dr. Ingram prescribed chemotherapy. Minot did not have the facilities for this treatment, and so Dr. Ingram said that he would send Ted to a hospital in Minneapolis. That was the nearest facility; he didn't want me to have to travel clear to Denver or Houston all by myself.

Ted was flown by Air Force Medical Air Lift in the middle of September. I drove down with Margaret, and we stayed at her sister's home. It was completely across the city of Minneapolis, but was a warm, friendly haven to come back to after long, trying days at the hospital.

They finally located the tumor at the base of Ted's brain. There was a little, short, fat German doctor who was in charge of the cancer ward. He insisted that Ted have brain surgery to relieve the pressure, warning him that he would die within days without it. Ted's face was swollen and his stomach distended greatly as part of the side effects of the long use of steroids, and by now he was quite disoriented. He did not know which way to turn to go to the dining room or the bathroom when he got to the door of his room. He was in a wheelchair most of the time. He could walk to the bathroom, which was right next door, but that was all.

One morning a Japanese doctor made rounds with the little German doctor. He returned alone later, to say that he felt Ted should know the risk of surgery. There was a very real possibility that Ted would be a "vegetable." He could go across the hall and down one door and see a young man, only twenty-six, who had been lying for five months, neither knowing or moving—just curled in a fetal ball. He said, "Fortunately, he has a temperature of one hundred five, and I hope he dies soon, for his sake and his family's." The boy did die the next day. His family told me that those five months were the most painful part to endure in losing their son.

Ted planned to call his sister Grace, who was a nurse, as he valued her professional opinion. He was going to call Ed, his minister brother, valuing his spiritual opinion. He even considered calling his parents to ask their opinion about risking brain surgery to relieve the pressure. Before I left him that night, I told him, "Ted, I love you and will take care of you if you should become a 'vegetable.' I don't want to lose you, but it is your life and you must choose. I will accept and stand by you whatever you decide."

When I returned the next morning, he said, "You don't have to say anything. I made up my own mind last night. If I called my family and asked their opinion and it turned out badly, they would be forever burdened with guilt because they suggested the wrong way. I decided that it is my life and I will choose how it will end.

"I want you to call Dr. Ingram and have him make arrangements for me to fly back to Minot. I want to go home and be near the kids. What is the use of going through the pain and sickness of major surgery to keep me alive four or five months, when it would be months of physical pain from the surgery, and emotional pain of being separated from the children? What is the value to live more months being away from all I love? I want to go home and be with Lorie, Jody, and Ruff. If I could choose, I would take Ruff out in the pasture, and we'd both die out there. I don't think that dog will want to live without me." I hastened to assure him that I didn't either!

As we were discussing this, the head nurse came in, and he told her of his battle trying to decide during the night. She said, "Ted, I have worked on this cancer ward for sixteen years, and believe me, you have chosen the better way. They might relieve the pressure on your brain long enough for you to die of lung cancer; but believe me, it is much easier to die of a brain tumor. You will simply sleep more and more, and finally not wake up. Go home—be with your children—love your family—you have chosen wisely!"

That afternoon I met the chief of social services in the hall. She asked how we could face Ted's impending death so calmly. According to her, all the nurses were talking about us; we were the main topic of conversation at every meeting and during lunch hours. I assured her that it wasn't because we were super-brave or courageous. Instead, our lives were totally committed to Jesus Christ. We trusted Him to decide what was best for us and to lead, not where we chose, but where He could use us. Not fully understanding, she wished us well, her eyes glistening with tears as she left.

I drove Ted to the Minneapolis airport early the next morning. Dr. Ingram had set things in motion to have him readmitted at the Minot hospital until I could drive the five hundred miles home and pick him up. Ted insisted on going home one more time. Fall had arrived, with her beautiful red and yellow leaves and hazy days. He wanted to be in our home as a family one more time and see all he loved and had worked for for so many years.

When I went to pick Ted up at the hospital in Minot, a corpsman stopped me as I went down the hall. He had been working in one of the wards earlier that morning when Ted went down the hall on his crutches, singing, "Oh, What a Beautiful Morning" at the top of his lungs. One of the ward patients complained, "What kind of fool would sing a song like that in a place like this?" The man in the bed across from him laughingly explained, "Oh, that must be Scheresky—only he could sing like that, knowing he's dying!"

We hurried home, and the children were waiting for us. Ruff was ecstatic, jumping and barking because his friend was home once again.

Sadly, Ted was only home two days when he became dreadfully ill, again not knowing who or where he was. We took him back to the hospital and were told that the doctors really thought he was dying that day. Again, with an adjustment in the Decadron, Ted pulled out of it one more time.

After a couple of weeks, he begged to go home just once more. Dr. Ingram hesitated, but Ted wouldn't take no for an answer, so he came home for what was to be his last visit. His sister Agnes flew from California to see him, and Viola and Grace came from Chicago to visit him over another weekend. When they arrived, he met them at the door and greeted them with smiles and hugs, but he had to go outside, even on his crutches, and get control of his emotions before he came back in.

When they left, we walked out to the gate. He kissed them goodbye, and we stood in their headlights with his arm around me, waving and smiling as they drove away. It was a very painful time for them all. Ted was the big brother and well loved. I am sure it was difficult for them to drive away, knowing they would never see him alive again.

The days were Indian summer: leaves yellow, red, and brown, fields ripe with harvest. Ted counselled Lorie about what to do when he was alone. As a family, we talked calmly about our future without him. He tried to give us his wisdom and knowledge, but it was simply too much, at least for me, to absorb. I should have been more aware of running a huge operation like the farm before I was left alone. But of course, I never dreamed such a task would be mine.

The days were golden and warm in the sun. The evenings were cool, and in the early mornings the grass was shiny with little drops of dew. It seemed that nature was putting on her best face for Ted. He slept more and more, but at least a couple of times a day he would walk slowly to the mailbox and back, with a detour to the chicken house.

It was no secret that I had always hated the chickens. I thought they were dirty, highly excitable, and dumb—and they knew of my distaste for them. I am convinced the feeling was mutual! Whenever I went to gather eggs, there were a select few who wouldn't get off their nests, and I would have to act brave and try to calmly reach under them. They would slowly turn their beady little eyes on me and look very disdainfully at me. Just as I grasped the egg, they would either peck me soundly or they would fly out in a flurry of feathers, straw, dust, and much loud squawking.

Nevertheless, they were Ted's friends. Every day he would sit on an upturned five-gallon pail and, putting his crutches on the ground beside him, he would talk to them as he always did. They would gather around him and a few would climb right up into his lap. He would smooth their feathers and have lengthy conversations with them in the warm, autumn afternoons of the autumn of his life.

I soon noticed when I bathed him that his legs were bruised and bleeding. He finally admitted that he was falling often. I hated to tell him that he shouldn't go out anymore, so I merely made it a point to go with him.

As the days passed, Ted started losing consciousness more and more. Often as he stood by the sink brushing his teeth or combing his hair, he would suddenly grab the doorpost and slide down it to the floor. One weekend the children had gone to church when he fell beside the refrigerator. I had to let him lie on the kitchen floor until Lorie got home to help me get him into bed. We wordlessly understood that his time was getting more limited; that he would soon have to return to the hospital.

Finally one evening Ted said, "You better call Mamma and Papa and tell them that I am not doing too well. They may want to come back again." They had come to see him, with his sister Carol in June, when he came home from the hospital the first time. Understandably this was a very difficult thing for them to accept. Their first son, one they loved with pride. To lose him in the prime of his life—my heart ached for them. I had let the other children decide how and when and how much to tell them, to spare them what pain they could, but now Ted told me that he was their child, and they deserved to know the truth. He wanted them to know it would not be much longer. It was a very difficult phone call to make.

While rubbing Ted's back with lotion, I discovered a lump as large as a baseball where the kidney had been removed. On the following Tuesday, during a checkup, I silently pointed to his back as he lay facing away from us on the examination table. Dr. Ingram excused himself and went out, returning with the chief of staff. They both shook their heads, but said nothing. Motioning me out into the hall, Dr. Ingram said, "Jean, it is time to bring him back. This is enough—you can't go on like this anymore. He'll fall more and more, and you simply cannot handle him. His right side is noticeably weaker. He soon won't be able to handle the crutches at all—that is the reason he is falling now." His kindness wrung my heart, as did the thought of bringing Ted back for the last time.

When I could speak, I told him that I would do whatever Ted wanted. We went back in to talk to him. Dr. Ingram explained gently that it was time to come back, but Ted begged for just one more weekend. He turned to me and said, "Can we make it a couple of more days, Honey?" I numbly nodded yes, and tears slipped down the faces of all three of us.

John helped Ted into the wheelchair, and, as busy as he was, he went down in the elevator to help me get him into the car. We talked on the way home about how good God had been to send this particular young man into our lives for this time.

7
A Passport to Peace

The day Ted left home for the last time it was cold and raw, with a biting wind. Ed and Jim had come early so Ted could talk with them and Lorie about what crops to put where and how to manage the rest of the farm.

The ambulance was waiting to go. Ed helped get the stretcher through the door, and I got into the ambulance with Ted. He smiled and waved cheerfully as we pulled away from the gate and left the three men standing there in that freezing wind with tears on all of their faces. Leaving our home with all of its hopes and dreams for the very last time was not the ordeal we had feared. We felt completely undergirded by God's love and strength.

The day Dr. Ingram had tried to convince Ted to come back to the hospital, Ted's main disagreement had been that he didn't want to be parted from me. Dr. Ingram promised he'd arrange for me to stay with him twenty-four hours a day. True to his word, when we arrived, we found the head nurse, Major Maley, had brought a cot from her own home and installed it beside Ted's bed. I slept there for the remaining days of Ted's life.

I will be forever grateful for the understanding and loving kindness which helped us through a very difficult time. All through these last confusing, anxious days, our greatest spiritual asset was our utterly complete consciousness of the actual presence of Jesus Christ in our lives.

Ted was eating very little by now, and the orderlies, the men in the kitchen, the corpsmen, and the nurses kept trying to tempt him with something special. Within days, his right side was partially paralyzed and he couldn't feed himself. He found this very humiliating. At first he sent me to the dime store for a rubber ball to squeeze, thinking he would work on those muscles and get his strength back. After two days, he sadly told me to throw it away.

The strain of those last two weeks was enormous; we expected him to die anytime. He slept more and more, and ate practically nothing.

One day Ted himself asked when his waiting would be over. The doctor kept telling him he had to be there for Thanksgiving—he promised to come and eat dinner with him.

November fifteenth was our wedding anniversary. When I woke up in the morning I kissed him and said, "Happy anniversary, darling!"

He stared at me vacantly, and slowly said, "Who are you?" I tried to explain, to see if I could bring our life into focus for him, but he started to cry, and said, "And who am I?"

I finally called the nurse, who kindly gave him a hypo and put him to sleep. When he wakened four hours later, he was himself. What a terrible day—how I thanked the Lord that he didn't go through more such times.

The days dragged by. His parents and our friends came, until he asked not to see anyone else but the family. It was too difficult, he said—not for him, but for those who had to say goodbye, knowing he was dying.

Thanksgiving finally arrived, and Dr. Ingram left his own family to come and see us. Ted ate exactly two bites of the huge tray of food that had been brought to him. The doctor took his hand and said, "See, Ted, I told you that you'd make it to Thanksgiving. Now you have to aim for Christmas!"

Ted smiled weakly and said, "No, Doc, I know I won't make it to Christmas. That is all right—this is enough. I want the Lord to take me home."

On Saturday morning his blood pressure dropped quickly to almost nothing. The nurse told me to call his family to come if they wished. They placed him on the VSI list. (Very Seriously Ill—not expected to live twenty-four hours.) The hospital chaplain was notified, but when he came, Ted did not respond to him. He kindly offered to call our pastor, who soon appeared. Ted opened his eyes and smiled, squeezing his hand when he prayed.

In the afternoon I called the children and told them that Daddy wasn't expected to live through the day. He had told them that he didn't want them to come and stand to watch him die. That was not a measure of their love. I left it up to them—they should choose. If they wished, they could come.

When our friends, Sam and Ruth, brought Jody to the hospital about four, I managed to rouse Ted. He took her hand, telling her to be a good girl, that he loved her, but to please go home—he wanted to spare her those last hours. Just after Jody left the room, Lorie came in and visited with his father for the last time. Jim and Diane finally took his parents home late in the evening. My heart broke for them as they kissed him goodbye and walked slowly out of the room.

That night, sitting beside the bed of my loved one, holding the dear hand that had worked so hard for me, that had never touched me in anger, but always with gentleness and love, that now was still and didn't respond to my touch—I thought my heart would break. I prayed I'd be a witness to God's ability to take me through such a difficult place.

I had been so busy with Ted's impending death I hadn't taken time to read my devotions that morning. As I sat alone after midnight, I read from Mrs. Cowman's book:

> A promise [is] given for hard places . . . not removal from the noise of the battle and the presence of our foes; but it means a shelter from the storm, a fortress amid the foe, a life preserved in the face of continual pressure.
>
> *Days of Heaven upon Earth*

> We often pray to be delivered from calamities; we even trust that we shall be; but we do not pray to be

> made what we should be, in the very presence of the calamities; to live amid them as long as they last, in the consciousness that we are held and sheltered by the Lord, and can therefore remain in the midst of them . . . .

Again and again through the long, endless night, my heart sang with joy that our mighty God was my personal Friend, and that He was able to keep me in the midst of that trial!

Toward morning, as the sky was turning pink with the dawn of a new day, I walked down to the end of the hall and looked out over the town. I can feel today what I felt that morning as I prayed, "Oh, Loving Father, I don't understand why You have let this happen. I cannot fathom why You would let a man of Ted's ability and consecration die. I can only trust You. You must have a plan of some kind. Use this long nightmare we have been through to help others. Please, I beg You, don't let this all be for nothing. I don't know what You can do with a middle-aged, tired, confused lady, but You've got one. I can't imagine what earthly use You can find for me—but I am Yours. Take the broken pieces of my life and make something useful of them."

I waited all through that day, but there was no change. Ed and Marge came in the evening. Ted was in a coma—we were simply waiting for the end.

After another long night of waiting, Ted was breathing very heavily. Dr. Ingram sent a corpsman in to wait with me. He was there only minutes when Ted's breathing became irregular. The corpsman ran to get the doctor and nurses.

While I was alone, I put my face next to his and said my goodbye, thanking him for the many years of happiness he had given to me, promising to meet him in God's new day. I kissed his dear, parched lips for the last time as the small army of the medical team arrived.

I stood there until he stopped breathing, then I quietly opened the door and slowly walked out into the hall.

After about five minutes, the doctor came out of Ted's room and walked over to where I stood leaning against the wall. He said, "Jean, I want you to know that I feel as badly as if my own brother had just died. I will never be the same doctor, the same husband, son, or father that I was before I met you and Ted and the witness of your lives through these last four months." How I thanked the Lord for being true to His promises and providing all that we needed.

Within the hour, Ed and Marge arrived and we made the necessary arrangements together. When we got home, I felt completely drained of all my strength. Since I hadn't slept for three nights, I went in to lie down. Ed said he would tell the folks, but I wanted to tell the children. They met the news with quiet courage. We had expected it for a long time. We couldn't help but be thankful that his long ordeal was over. He had welcomed death as a passport to peace and rest.

The funeral loomed ahead of us. There really isn't any way to escape the pain and emptiness—it simply has to be lived through. You know that the hours and days will eventually pass—on silent, wooden wheels, it is true—but they do pass.

Ted had asked me to call our minister and friend to come to the hospital to discuss his funeral. He was adamant that nothing but songs of hope and joy be sung. He said to use the taped music that he loved to listen to at home. He didn't want to ask any of our friends to sing; it would be too difficult for them. He didn't want to cause anyone pain. He asked that there be no committal service at the cemetery. He was concerned for his parents and wanted to spare all of us any avoidable pain or anguish.

Walking into the church the day of the funeral was one of the hard spots. It was packed: inside, outside, downstairs, the balcony, and the gymnasium next door were filled.

During the service, both ministers spoke of Ted's consistent Christian witness. Throughout all the long months of his illness, he never gave up his belief that God makes no mistakes, and he died with great serenity. He refused to be defeated. They reminded us it is not the number of years that we live that is significant; it is the quality of the life we live—whether the years be many or few—and the courage with which we face those years, that count.

They spoke of Ted's pain at leaving his family, and his desire to be there to encourage his nieces and nephews to love and serve Jesus Christ, too. Someday we would all be together again. One of the songs Ted had chosen was:

> Meet me in Heaven, we'll sing songs together,
> Meet me at the Saviour's feet.
>
> Meet me in Heaven, we'll join hands together,
> Brothers and sisters we'll be there.

Ted had made me promise I would not walk down the aisle with my head bowed in defeat, but to prove that God *was* able to do as He promised; to take us through the valley of death victoriously. I didn't say easily, or painlessly, or without despair, but victoriously—and He did!

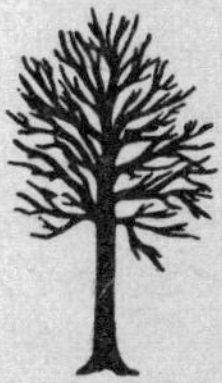

8

It's O.K. to Cry!

Facing death is difficult at best, and sometimes it is nearly impossible to understand or cope with as an adult. This is true to a much greater degree for children, especially those in their teen years. They are "too big to cry," and I am sure that part of our two children's inability to express their grief was their father's admonition to "be brave and help Mother." They were so brave that it became pitiful, and my heart broke for them, over and over again.

They knew that everyone was watching to see how they took it, and we all wanted to be a witness to God's ability to see us through such a long, dark valley. Jody and Lorie were strong, stalwart, and brave, but I feel they tried too hard, and suffered for it.

I was surprised to read Jody's term paper for her English class the spring after Ted's death. I doubt that she would have given it to me to read, but she was sick with the flu and had to ask me to type it for her.

The title was "Chemotherapy—Yes or No." I was amazed as I read:

> My father just died of cancer. He had to choose whether to have chemotherapy or not. He chose not to have it—he wanted to come home and spend what time he had left of his life near us. He could have possibly lived a few months longer, but be sick and far away from home. He chose more quality and less quantity. I think he chose wisely.

She did an excellent job on the paper. She had written to the doctor at the Mayo Clinic. The paper was intelligent, objective, factual, and it seemingly didn't bother her to tell about it. I was very proud of her and how grown-up she was. Several months later, all her braveness caught up with her.

While counselling at our church camp in the summer, she woke up crying one morning and couldn't stop for a day and a half. I asked her if she had heard a song that reminded her of Daddy, or a sermon on heaven? What had triggered it?

"Mother, I don't know what caused it. When I woke up that morning, I honestly felt worse than the day he died or the day of the funeral. I just missed him so much that all the tears I haven't shed for all these months spilled over. Once they got started, I couldn't seem to turn them off."

Shannon, Jody's best friend, frightened when she saw the storm of tears was not going to stop, ran for the camp nurse. How thankful I was that particular lady was there. She had watched her baby die, and, of course, was very understanding, sympathetic, and supportive of Jody's grief.

I finally sat down with both of the children and explained that *it's O.K. to cry!* Tears are a normal part of grief. They are nothing to be ashamed of. It is best to try to control yourself, to a degree. Throwing yourself on the floor and kicking and screaming will get you nothing but a sore throat and skinned heels, but don't feel ashamed or embarrassed to cry.

Even today, my tears come unbidden at a special song or a memory, but they need not be choked back and swallowed.

Jody and I had a long talk one day as I was driving her back to school after a home leave. I pointed out to her that Daddy was a wonderful man. He was an unusual father; teasing, fun, loving, helpful, kind. He was *worth* crying over.

We had lost an important, needed, wonderful part of our lives when he died. Tears shed over our loss were not a sign of being a baby—they were part of the healing process from our grief and sorrow that we no longer had him as part of our lives and our family.

We discovered God did not just wave a magic wand and dissolve our grief, but He quieted our questioning, and fear, with His love.

He has given me peace when the house is so empty, and release from numbness, bewilderment, and despair. From Him has come strength to live my life without Ted with meaning and purpose. A treasured friend asked me, "What did you talk about? How could you bear to actually *talk* about losing all your hopes and dreams or facing the future alone? I wouldn't know what to say if my husband was facing death, and I was facing life without him!"

The first, very natural reaction is to ignore it and hope it will go away. But it won't!

Each of us is made differently. What was right for me might not be right for you. I would not presume to set down any rules that say what has to be said or done, I am sharing what worked for us in facing this problem.

Ted was an eternal optimist—he honestly tried not to worry about problems. He did his best and trusted the Lord to do what he couldn't in any situation.

For Ted, the hardest part of the whole seven months he was dying was to finally accept that God wasn't going to heal him, or at least give him another couple of years. God *does* answer all of our prayers, sometimes not the way we want—but answer He does! Sometimes the answer is *no*. Just as it is difficult for our children to understand our *no* to their childish wishes, sometimes it is nearly impossible to understand and accept God's *no* to our prayers and pleas.

We had two choices. We could have ignored the situation and pretended that it wasn't really happening, or we could face it, accept it, and talk about it. This is the path we chose together.

I am grateful that we had happy memories to share. I am sure it would be painful if our life together had been full of fighting and misery. The load of guilt for memories would indeed become heavy. If this is true for you, I can only admonish you to ask each other for loving forgiveness and make what time you have left to share a sweet, caring, sharing time together.

The very most important thing is to *be honest* with each other. Don't be afraid to admit that you are frightened, or hate the thought of being left alone, or having your financial future looking desolate.

Unless you are a perfect paragon of virtue, are independently wealthy, and are childless, you *will* have these feelings of uncertainty and worry and concern. *Share them.*

Because of his illness, at first I didn't want to worry Ted with my concern for the future. In fact, to be perfectly honest, I tried not to think about it at all. One afternoon I was sitting beside him, fingers locked in his, my head laid on the side of the bed in total weariness.

"Jean," he said, "I have loved and taken care of you for over twenty years, and I had planned to do so all of your life. I know it must be frightening to think of being left alone. Please tell me what scares you the most. Let me help you as long as I can. Some things I will not be able to solve for you, but let me suggest and find solutions where I can, as long as I am able."

This became a learning and sharing time for us as we talked many hours about problems that might arise, about possible solutions, about alternatives, and the possibility of failure for some of those plans. He counselled me to do as we had in the past—to do the very best we could and leave what we couldn't solve to Jesus Christ. We are His, and all of these seemingly insurmountable problems become His, too.

Next to being honest is being *patient,* not only with each other, but with others. Many people want to help, and blunder in doing so, but all mean kindly. After weeks and months of weariness, I blundered, too.

God is gentle and kind and does supply us with His strength and courage, but He doesn't make over our personality, and with one fell swoop transform our faults and failures, endowing us with halos.

When an illness goes on and on—day after dreary, weary days—you can become terribly tired physically, as well as emotionally drained. Being loving and patient can become an effort as you struggle to keep your courage and strength at a high level.

Today, I hear couples that bicker and are impatient with each other who are *not* facing death. My heart always aches, thinking, "Oh, don't waste your time together fighting over inconsequential things! In the light of eternity, does it really matter?"

Don't waste your time together. Enjoy each other, your family, your health. Take time for each other. Listen to each other—really listen! Don't forget to take time to share life with each other. Don't put off enjoying life—you may not have that life to share together.

It is not always easy to find time to share with each other and with your children, but I would admonish you to not only find time, but *make* time for your family.

God expects us to serve Him fully and constantly, but not at the expense of neglecting the family that He has given to you for a charge. Don't let yourself be that busy. Don't neglect to share the worries and seemingly foolish fears and triumphs. These are important years for them: Share them, or risk losing them. Make happy memories—what if your family life was to end tomorrow? Are you really satisfied with the memories you would leave?

Take time—*make time*—to be kind, patient, and loving with each other. We have no assurance of tomorrow. Do not think, "It couldn't happen to me!" It could!

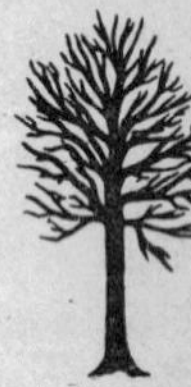

9

"Now We See Through a Glass, Darkly . . ."

I still do not know the reason *why,* but I am not looking for it! I still have complete confidence that God has a plan for each of His children, and I accept what He has allowed to come into my life. I still do not understand, and being very honest, I confess I do not like it! But I have seen and felt and known God's working in my life. I know that all of my tomorrows are His and I trust Him to lead me in the future, as He has in the past. It was not an easy path He led us down, but the safe journey through the dark valley was made possible by His unfailing love and presence in our lives.

He does not lead me year by year
  Nor even day by day.
But step by step my path unfolds;
  My Lord directs my way.

Tomorrow's plans I do not know,
  I only know this minute;
But He will say, "This is the way,
  By faith, now walk ye in it."

And I am glad that it is so.
  Today's enough to bear,
And when tomorrow comes, His grace
  Shall far exceed its care.

What need to worry then, or fret;
  The God who gave His Son
Holds all my moments in His hand
  And gives them, one by one.

BARBARA C. RYBERG

He promised He would never leave me nor forsake me. *He didn't!*

He promised that even though I walked through the valley of the shadow of death, I need fear no evil. *I didn't!*

He promised His Grace would be sufficient. *It was!*

He promised to be my refuge and strength. *He is!*

He promised to go before me. *He has and He will!*

I have proved God's promises are true. . . . Let Him prove them in your life, too.